I0423901

Anti-Inflammatory Diet

The Ultimate Guide to Looking 10
Years Younger, Having More Energy
and Less Pain

James P. Kaplan

Legal & Disclaimer

Legal & Disclaimer

The information contained in this book is not designed to replace or take the place of any form of medicine or professional medical advice. The information in this book has been provided for educational and entertainment purposes only.

The information contained in this book has been compiled from sources deemed reliable, and it is accurate to the best of the Author's knowledge; however, the Author cannot guarantee its accuracy and validity and cannot be held liable for any errors or omissions. Changes are periodically made to this book. You must consult your doctor or get professional medical advice before using any of the suggested remedies, techniques, or information in this book.

Upon using the information contained in this book, you agree to hold harmless the Author from and against any damages, costs, and expenses, including any legal fees potentially resulting from the application of any of the information provided by this guide. This disclaimer applies to any damages or injury caused by the use and application, whether directly or indirectly, of any advice or information presented, whether for breach of contract, tort, negligence, personal injury, criminal intent, or under any other cause of action.

You agree to accept all risks of using the information presented inside this book. You need to consult a professional medical practitioner in order to ensure you are both able and healthy enough to participate in this program.

Table of Contents

Smoothie & Shake Recipes..

Conclusion

Introduction

The anti-inflammatory diet doesn't have a catchy name like most of the other diets out on the market. It doesn't promise that you'll lose 10 pounds in 10 days. More than a diet, it's a life-long eating plan.

It has become clear that long term inflammation is the main cause for many serious illness. Everyone knows the signs of inflammation on the skin; local redness, heat, swelling and pain. It shows that the body is working to repair itself by bringing more blood (nourishment) and immune activity to the site of infection or injury. However, when that inflammation hangs on or occurs where no injury or infection is located, it can damage the tissues and cause illness.

Supporters of this diet believe that it can reduce the risk of heart disease as well as keeping current heart problems from worsening. It can reduce the level of triglycerides in the blood, blood pressure and ease the symptoms of arthritis. Following this diet can make losing weight easier, and even has the potential to slow down the aging process as well.

While this diet can help with the problems mentioned here, scientific research is still being performed to determine just how beneficial this eating plan can be for many other diseases.

Within the pages of this book you will learn what the anti-inflammatory lifestyle is so that you can determine if it is for you, what foods you can eat and which you should avoid to prevent further inflammation and some recipes to get you started.

What Is Inflammation?

One thing that should always be remembered when thinking about inflammation is that inflammation is *not* a bad thing. When you are ill or injured, your immune system sends in the cavalry. White blood cells and excess blood floods the area of injury or infection; the white blood cells to fight off any intruders and the blood to wash it away. Because a specific area is getting more attention like this, you will most likely experience swelling and redness, heat and varying levels of pain. This is a perfectly normal response of your body to promote healing. Unfortunately, that isn't always the case.

Inflammation as described in the preceding paragraph is considered acute inflammation; this is what is considered good inflammation. However, when your immune system attacks healthy body tissues it becomes chronic which can lead to more and worsening diseases. Chronic inflammation often doesn't come with any symptoms until one of these other diseases finally begins to affect your life. For example, inflamed airways can cause an asthma attack, excess fluids in joints can lead to arthritis and the affect inflammation has on insulin resistance can worsen diabetes.

The bottom line is that inflammation helps your body to defend itself against infection and illness from injury or bacterial/viral attack. Unfortunately, it can also occur on a chronic basis causing other diseases.

What Causes Inflammation?

Lifestyle and dietary factors can all promote inflammation, especially if you don't alter those lifestyles and dietary factors.

Inflammation Triggers

- Sugar. Consuming a lot of sugary foods is particularly bad since it can lead to insulin resistance, diabetes and weight gain.
- Refined carbohydrates. White bread and pasta made from refined flour also contributes to inflammation, insulin resistance and weight gain.
- Processed foods. These contain trans fat which have also been shown to damage the cells lining your arteries.
- Vegetable oils. These are used in many processed foods. Consuming them on a regular basis can cause an omega-6 to omega-3 imbalance.
- Alcohol. Excess consumption can cause inflammation in the liver which can effect insulin use. Alcohol is also very high in sugar.
- Processed meat. Additives that prevent spoilage are known to cause inflammation. Processed meats also contain high amounts of trans fats and sugar to make them flavorful.
- Lack of exercise. A sedentary lifestyle is a major non-dietary factor that promotes inflammation.
- Excess weight. Extra fat cells in the body causes stress on healthy tissue. Over time that stress will cause increased inflammation.

- Stress and anxiety. Outside stressors cause a reaction called fight-or-flight which causes your body to produce increased levels of cortisol which is known to increase fat production and storage.
- Pollution. When your body takes in polluted air and water, your immune system is mobilized to fight off the irritating particles. However, often the pollution – especially air pollution – overwhelms your body's resistance and the white blood cells go into an offensive mode rather than defensive. This causes inflammation in the lung tissue which can lead to lung diseases.

How to Reduce Inflammation?

There are several ways to reduce chronic inflammation in your body. Reducing that chronic inflammation can also decrease the chance of developing worse diseases or possibly reverse those diseases altogether.

If you want to reduce inflammation, you can eat fewer inflammatory foods and consume more anti-inflammatory foods. You will find a listing later on in this book to let you know which foods you should enjoy and which you should avoid or reduce. You should base your new diet on whole, nutrient-dense foods and avoid anything processed.

Foods high in antioxidants will help to reduce inflammation. Antioxidants reduce the levels of free radicals in your system. If free radicals are not kept under control it can lead to inflammation.

You should try to eat a diet balanced in protein, carbs and fats with each meal while still being sure to get enough vitamins, minerals, fiber and water as well. Low-carb diets such as the Mediterranean diet and The Zone have been shown to help reduce inflammation but those can sometimes be expensive to follow. Vegetarian diets are also known to reduce inflammation.

The bottom line is that you can choose a balanced diet, cut out processed foods and boost consumption of anti-inflammatory and antioxidant-rich foods to reduce inflammation in your body.

Why Follow the Anti-Inflammatory Diet?

Eating is something you do every day, multiple times a day. It is known that what you eat has both an immediate and a long term effect on your body. This is why so many diet proponents – no matter what diet they support – insist that their diet will cause a certain reaction from your body to help you live better if you follow it.

Just like with a diet you follow to lose weight or reduce cholesterol, your diet can be the key in preventing and managing chronic inflammation in your body.

The one thing that many people worry about when they choose to follow a new dietary lifestyle. That is that they will always be hungry while following the diet and that they won't be able to enjoy some of their favorite foods. The thing about this lifestyle is that you won't be hungry since your caloric intake isn't as restrictive as most traditional diets tend to be. Not only will you not be hungry, you won't even have to give up all of your favorite foods.

The anti-inflammatory diet in addition to a good exercise program and adequate sleep time will help you improve many aspects of your life.

- reduced symptoms of arthritis
- improvement in the symptoms of inflammatory bowel syndrome, lupus and other autoimmune diseases
- weight loss
- decreased risk of heart disease, depression, diabetes, cancer and many other diseases
- fewer inflammatory markers in your blood

- blood sugar, cholesterol and triglyceride levels will be closer to normal
- improvement in moods
- increased energy

Following the anti-inflammatory diet and altering your lifestyle to accommodate the new routine can help reduce the risk of you developing many diseases.

Tips & Tricks

It has become very clear that chronic inflammation – mainly caused by obesity – is the root cause of many serious diseases. As the number of people diagnosed as obese grows, so will the occurrences of heart disease, Alzheimer's disease and many cancers grow.

Doctors and nutritionists know that proper nourishment and immune activity is the foundation of your body's healing response. Unfortunately, when inflammation serves no purpose it damages your body at the cellular level and causes illnesses.

Lack of exercise, stress, exposure to toxins and genetic predisposition can all contribute to chronic inflammation but the foods you choose also plays a very large role. When you learn how certain foods influence the inflammatory process, you can develop a strategy for reducing your risk for long-term diseases.

Tips to Following the Diet

- Shoot for variety.
- Eat as much fresh food as possible.
- Stop eating processed foods and fast food.
- Eat a lot of fruits and vegetables.

Most adults need to take in between 2,000 and 3,000 calories per day though women and less active people generally need fewer calories than men. If you eat the appropriate number of calories for your level of activity then your weight should not fluctuate very much. If you are wanting to lose weight while controlling inflammation, you will want to reduce your caloric intake each day but be sure not to starve yourself either. You will want to consume between 40 and 50 percent of your calories from good carbohydrates, 30 percent from good fats and 20 to 30 percent from lean proteins. You want to include a serving of each at every meal.

Carbohydrates

- Adult women on a 2,000 calorie diet will consume between 160 and 200 grams of carbohydrates on a daily basis.
- Adult men on a 2,000 calorie diet will consume between 240 and 300 grams of carbohydrates on a daily basis.
- All of your carbohydrates should come from less refined and less processed foods. Most fruits and vegetables contain carbohydrates so you should focus on those for your carb consumption. However, you do need to watch the glycemic load of those fruits and vegetables.
- Restrict your consumption of bread, chips, pretzels, cookies, etc. These foods contain high amounts of processed flour and sugar.
- Eat whole grains like brown rice and bulgur wheat since the grain is intact. These are better for you than whole wheat flour products which has the same glycemic load as white flour products.
- Include beans, squash and sweet potatoes in your diet.
- Eat pasta in moderation. It should be cooked al dente.
- Avoid anything made with high fructose corn syrup.

Fats

- As with carbohydrates, men and women will consume slightly different amounts of fats from nutritious sources.
- On a 2,000 calorie diet, about 600 calories will come from fats. This amount is about 67 grams. You will want to take in more monounsaturated fats than saturated or polyunsaturated fats. The ratio is 1:2:1.
- Strictly avoid tran-fats.
- Eat less butter, cream, high-fat cheese, unskinned chicken and fatty meats as well as items made with palm kernel oil.
- Extra-virgin olive oil should be used as your main cooking oil.
- You will want to avoid regular safflower and sunflower oils, corn oil, cottonseed oil and any mixed vegetable oil.
- Margarine, vegetable shortening and any product with those listed in the ingredients should be strictly avoided.
- If hydrogenated or partially hydrogenated oils appear in the ingredients, that product should also be removed from your diet.
- Include avocados and nuts or nut butters in your diet.
- Omega-3 fatty acids are essential for reducing inflammation. Eat salmon, sardines, herring, black cod, hemp seeds and flax seeds. You can also take a fish oil supplement; a daily dosage of 2 to 3 grams is suggested.

Protein

- Daily protein intake should be between 80 and 120 grams on a 2,000 calorie diet. You will need to eat less protein if you have kidney or liver problems, allergies or an autoimmune disease.
- Reduce your consumption of beef, pork and poultry. Fish, high quality natural cheese and yogurt should be used in place of animal proteins.
- Eat more vegetable proteins such as beans and soy products. You will want to become familiar with the whole-soy foods available in your area.

Fiber and Water

- You need to eat about 40 grams of fiber each day.
- Increase consumption of fruit, beans and whole grains.
- Ready-made cereals are good sources of fiber but you must read the labels to be sure you are getting at least 5 grams of bran in every serving. Also check the label for those ingredients you should strictly avoid.
- You want to drink pure water or drinks that are mostly water all day. Tea, sparkling water with lemon, unsweetened drinks are allowed.
- Avoid any drink that contains any kind of artificial sweetener since those chemicals can contribute to inflammation.
- Use bottled water or purchase a purifier for your home.

What to Eat & Avoid

When your body is in an inflammatory state, what you eat can make a difference. Some foods increase inflammation which can trigger other chronic conditions but others help reduce inflammation. Below, you will find a listing of food items or ingredients in pre-packaged foods that you should avoid as well as a listing of foods that work to reduce inflammation.

Inflammatory Ingredients & Foods

1. Sugar. You might find it difficult to resist desserts, chocolate bars, soda and even fruit juice. However, it has been found that processed sugar can trigger the release of inflammatory cytokines. Cytokines are substances that are secreted by cells of the immune system; the most commonly known is human growth hormone. These cytokines have an effect on many other cells in your body. Sugar goes by a lot of different names so watch for any word ending in -ose, such as fructose and sucrose on ingredient labels.

2. Saturated Fats. According to the National Cancer Institute, pizza and cheese are the biggest sources of saturated fats in an average American diet. Several studies state that saturated fat consumption triggers inflammation in fat cells stored in your body. Besides pizza and cheese, other culprits include red meat, full-fat dairy, pasta and grain-based desserts.

3. Trans Fats. Researchers at the Harvard School of Public Health have been sounding the alarm about trans fats since the early 1990s. Trans fats are known to trigger inflammation systemically rather than just locally in your body. Trans fats are found in fast food and other fried foods, frozen breakfast products, processed snack items, crackers, cookies, donuts and most stick margarines. You should avoid any foods that include hydrogenated oils on the ingredient labels.

4. Omega-6 Fatty Acids. These are essential fatty acids that your body needs for normal growth and development. However, you need a healthy balance between Omega-6 and Omega-3 fatty acids. Consuming too many Omega-6s can trigger inflammation in your

body. These fatty acids are found in several types of oils; such as corn, safflower, sunflower, grapeseed, peanut, soy and vegetable. Mayonnaise and other commercial salad dressings also contain Omega-6 fatty acids.

5. Refined Carbohydrates. Products containing white flour, white rice, white potatoes and many cereals are made of refined carbs. Scientific American has stated that processed carbohydrates are the main reason for the rising rate of obesity and other chronic illnesses – even over fats! Refined carbohydrates are also called high glycemic index foods which stimulate inflammation.

6. MSG. Mono-sodium glutamate is a flavor enhancer added to foods and is most commonly found in pre-packaged Asian food and soy sauce. However, it has also been added to fast foods, canned soup and soup mixes, salad dressings and deli meats. This chemical not only triggers inflammation but also affects the health of your liver.

7. Gluten & Casein. These are proteins found in dairy and wheat which also promote inflammation. If you are unlucky enough to suffer from arthritis as well as celiac disease or dairy intolerance then the inflammatory effect will be compounded. Gluten is found in wheat, barley, rye and any foods made with those grains while casein is found in whey protein products.

8. Aspartame. This ingredient is an intense artificial sweetener found in more than 4,000 products worldwide. Not only does it have no nutritional value, it is also a neurotoxin which affects the brain. Whether you are sensitive to this chemical or not, your immune

system reacts to the foreign substance by attacking the chemical. This in turn triggers and inflammatory response in your digestive tract.

9. Alcohol. Alcohol is a large burden on your liver. If you drink more than 1 or 2 ounces of hard liquor, 10 ounces of wine or 24 ounces of beer it can weaken the way your liver functions and disrupt other multi-organ interactions. This causes more severe inflammation since the alcohol confuses every cell in your body. Either eliminate alcohol entirely from your diet or strictly moderate its consumption.

10. Dairy. Milk is for making calves gain weight quickly. Humans do not really require milk, we drink it because it tastes good. Researchers with the Harvard School of Public Health have found that bone strength does not come from drinking milk or consuming other dairy products but from plant foods that contain calcium. In fact, dairy is highly inflammatory for most people. Oddly enough, the more processed – skimmed – doesn't make milk healthier at all. It only makes it more inflammatory by concentrating the dairy proteins and sugars.

11. Tropical Fruits. Since they have a higher fructose content than most other fruits, you should moderate your consumption of tropical fruits. However, if you have diabetes you should limit them to once a week. Many people eat bananas because they are a wonderful source of potassium but many other fruits and vegetables also contain high levels of potassium.

12. Peanuts. Like milk, peanuts are also a common allergen. Allergies set off all kinds of inflammatory responses in your body while it tries to fight off the foreign substances. Peanuts are also prone to mold and

fungus growth which will also result in your body producing an inflammatory response.

13. Seasoning Mixes. Commercially made seasoning mixes are a short cut you may have used all your life. However, they usually contain artificial coloring, high amounts of sugar and various preservatives. All of these are known to cause inflammation.

14. Iodized Salt. While not harmful on its own, sodium is naturally found with other valuable minerals like potassium, calcium and magnesium. The iodizing process removes most of those minerals and replaces them with chlorine, which is toxic. Unrefined salt, such as sea salt, is a better choice and actually tastes better.

Cutting back on foods that promote inflammation, eating more fruits and vegetables, switching to fish for protein and consuming more Omega-3 foods will make a great difference in your inflammation symptoms.

Anti-inflammatory Foods

1. Whole Grains. You want to eat more whole grains to increase your fiber intake. Whole grains are known to help reduce inflammation. They are also known to have a lower glycemic index to keep your glucose levels down.

2. Berries & Tart Cherries. In general fruit is high in antioxidants. Berries in particular contain healthy polyphenols and anthocyanins which help to reduce inflammation.

3. Olive Oil. It is delicious, is good for both cold and hot uses and contains healthy oleic acid. Oleic acid reduces blood pressure, helps you burn fat and protects cells from free radicals.

4. Cruciferous Vegetables. Vegetables from the cabbage family contain most of the nutrients your body needs to work properly. They also contain antioxidants which helps to protect cells from the inflammation caused by free radicals. Below is a list of the vegetables in the cruciferous family.

   - Arugula
   - Bok Choi
   - Broccoli
   - Broccoli Rabe
   - Broccoli Romanesco
   - Brussels Sprouts
   - Cabbage
   - Cauliflower

- Chinese Broccoli
- Chinese Cabbage
- Collard Greens
- Daikon
- Horseradish
- Kale
- Kohlrabi
- Komatsuna
- Mustard – seeds and leaves
- Radish
- Rutabaga
- Turnips – roots and greens
- Wasabi
- Watercress

5. Fatty Fish. Cold-water fish like salmon, mackerel and sardines contain Omega-3 fatty acids which are known to have a significant anti-inflammatory effect if eaten 3-4 times a week.

6. Tomatoes. Tomatoes are high in lycopene which is another antioxidant that is thought to reduce inflammation in the lungs as well as other places in the body. Despite being a nightshade vegetable, there are no studies stating that nightshades cause inflammation.

7. Peppers. These also contain antioxidants – Vitamin C, in this case. Hot peppers also contain capsaicin which not only reduces

inflammation but is also a lipophilic chemical. This means that it increases the metabolism to help burn fat.

8. Leafy Greens. These foods contain an abundance of healthy compounds your body needs including Vitamin E, calcium, iron and several phytonutrients that help to reduce inflammation.

   - Romaine
   - Green Leaf Lettuce
   - Butterhead Lettuce
   - Swiss Chard
   - Spinach
   - Dandelion Greens
   - Red Clover
   - Plantain
   - Chickweed

9. Apples. Like most other fruits, apples contain healthy phytonutrients that help protect cells against premature aging.

10. Nuts. Nearly all nuts contain antioxidants which are key components in helping your body to fight inflammation. Walnuts are high in Omega-3 fatty acids while almonds and macadamia nuts contain large amounts of oleic acid. Except for peanuts, most nuts and their oils and butters are considered healthy fats.

11. Garlic & Onions. Both contain the antioxidant quercetin which naturally inhibits the release of histamine.

12. Soy & Soybeans. Soy foods contain large amounts of vegetable proteins as well as isoflavones which is thought to reduce inflammation. You want to avoid highly processed soy since it might contain additives. Check the labels of your tofu and soy milk to be sure you aren't choosing ones with additives and preservatives that could increase inflammation.
13. Ginger & Turmeric. These two spices are often found in Indian food. Turmeric contains curcumin which is particularly potent in fighting off inflammation.
14. Carrots. Rich in beta-carotene, carrots help reduce free radicals in your body.
15. Low-fat Dairy. While dairy promotes inflammation, high-quality and low-fat dairy products like cheese and yogurt are excellent sources of protein, calcium and probiotics.
16. Beets. Beets are no only colorful, they are also packed with Vitamin C, large amounts of fiber and lots of phytonutrients.
17. Winter Squash. While winter squash has always been recognized as an important source of carotenoids, it is only recently that research has documented that winter squash is a key food for getting these antioxidants. Winter squash is the primary food source for alpha- and beta-carotene – even better than carrots! It also contains lutein, zeaxanthin and beta-cryptoxanthin which are also healthy carotenoids.

   ◦ Ambercup

   ◦ Buttercup

   ◦ Hubbard

- Kabocha

- Turban

- Cushaw – a winter crook-necked squash

- Butternut

- Acorn

- Delicata

- Spaghetti

- Sweet Dumpling

- Sugar Loaf

- Pumpkin

18. Beans & Legumes. This is particularly important if you will be cutting out a great deal of your animal protein. Beans and legumes contain high amounts of vegetable protein as well as fiber.

19. Sweet Potatoes. While considered a carbohydrate, sweet potatoes also contain fiber, antioxidants and beta-carotene.

20. Tea. White, green and oolong tea are full of phytonutrients and flavonoids which helps to reduce inflammation. They also taste really good so you don't get bored with just drinking water all day.

Anti-inflammatory Supplements

If you find it difficult to get as much Omega-3 or other vitamins, minerals and phytonutrients, you can supplement your meals with a daily regimen of pills as well.

- Omega-3
- Vitamin C
- Vitamin E
- Borage or Starflower Oil
- Bioflavonoids
- Curcumin – aka Turmeric supplements
- Boswelia, Black Willow and Licorice
- Milk Thistle
- Co-enzyme Q10
- Zinc, Manganese & Selenium – required with most of the above to be absorbed properly.

Breakfast Recipes

Gingerbread Oatmeal

The key ingredient in helping to reduce inflammation is Omega-3 fatty acids. However, getting enough on a daily basis can be difficult. This oatmeal tastes wonderful and will give you half of your daily requirement of Omega-3s – without the salmon! Makes 4 servings.

Ingredients

- 4 c water
- 1c steel cut oats
- 1 ½ tbsp ground cinnamon
- ¼ tsp ground coriander
- 1 tsp ground cloves
- ¼ tsp ground ginger
- ¼ tsp ground allspice
- ⅛ tsp ground nutmeg
- ¼ tsp ground cardamom
- Maple syrup to taste

Directions

1. Combine oats and spices.
2. Cook oats according to package instructions.
3. When finished cooking, add maple syrup to taste.

Rhubarb & Ginger Muffins

Ginger is good but when you used crystallized ginger, it jumps to a level you may not have considered before. Combine it with tart rhubarb and these quick and easy muffins will become one of your favorite breakfast items. Makes 8 muffins.

Ingredients

- ½ c almond meal
- ¼ c raw sugar
- 2 tbsp crystallized ginger, finely chopped
- 1 tbsp flax seed meal
- ½ c buckwheat flour
- ¼ c fine brown rice flour
- 2 tbsp arrowroot powder
- 2 tsp baking powder
- ½ tsp ground cinnamon
- ½ tsp ground ginger
- ⅛ tsp high-quality sea salt
- 1 c fresh rhubarb, finely sliced
- 1 apple, peeled, cored and finely diced
- ⅓ c + 1 tbsp almond milk
- ¼ c olive oil
- 1 large egg
- 1 tsp vanilla extract

Directions

1. Preheat oven to 350 degrees.

2. Grease or line 8 standard sized muffin tin cavities.

3. In a large bowl, sift together almond meal, sugar, ground spices, flax seed meal and baking powder.

4. Add chopped ginger, rhubarb and apple. Stir to coat each piece.

5. In a small bowl, whisk together milk, egg, oil and vanilla.

6. Add wet mixture to dry mixture and stir until just combined.

7. Divide batter evenly between the muffin cavities.

8. Bake for 20-25 minutes until golden around the edges. When a toothpick inserted in the center comes out clean, it is done.

9. Remove from the oven and allow to cool in the pan for 5 minutes before turning out on a wire rack to finish cooling.

10. Enjoy warm or at room temperature. Store in an air tight container for 2 to 3 days or freeze for up to 1 week.

Buckwheat & Ginger Granola

This granola is wonderful served with coconut yogurt and fresh berries, mixed into a smoothie or sprinkled over stewed fruit as well. Makes a large container.

Ingredients

- 2 c steel cut oats
- 1 c buckwheat
- 1 c sunflower seeds
- 1 c pumpkin seeds

- 1 ½ c pitted dates
- 1 c unsweetened applesauce
- 6 tbsp coconut oil
- 4 tbsp unsweetened cocoa powder
- 4 tsp fresh ginger, peeled and finely grated

Directions

1. Preheat oven to 350 degrees.
2. In a large bowl, combine oats, buckwheats and seeds. Stir well.
3. In a small saucepan, melt coconut oil. When melted, add applesauce and dates. Simmer for 5 minutes until dates are soft.
4. Add ginger.
5. When dates are soft, pour contents of saucepan into a blender with cocoa powder. Blend until smooth.
6. Pour wet mixture over dry mixture and stir until well coated.
7. Grease one or two baking trays with coconut oil. Spread granola out on trays.
8. Bake for about 45 minutes. After 15 minutes, remove from oven and stir before returning trays to oven. Stir granola every 5-10 minutes for the remaining time to prevent burning.
9. When granola is crispy, remove from oven and allow to cool completely. Store in an air tight container for about 1 month.

Cinnamon & Walnut Pancakes

You probably thought you couldn't have pancakes when following an anti-inflammatory diet, didn't you? Well, guess what, these are low carb and low calorie and guaranteed not to cause inflammation. Coconut flour is an excellent tool to fight inflammation and the walnuts are a great source of Omega-3 as well.

Ingredients

- 4 eggs, room temperature
- 1 c coconut milk
- 2 tsp vanilla extract
- 1 tbsp raw honey
- ½ c walnuts, soaked, dried and chopped
- ½ c coconut flour
- 1 tsp baking soda
- ½ tsp sea salt
- ½ tsp cinnamon
- coconut oil for cooking

Directions

1. Preheat griddle over medium low heat.
2. In a small bowl, beat eggs until frothy and well broken down.
3. Add milk, vanilla and honey.
4. In a separate bowl, combine coconut flour, baking soda, cinnamon and sea salt. Whisk to combine.
5. Add wet mixture into dry mixture until all flour is incorporated.

6. Add walnuts. Mix to combine.
7. Grease griddle with coconut oil.
8. Ladle out batter onto griddle and let cook. Spread batter out so it doesn't mound in the center. Pancakes should be about 2-3 inches in diameter and slightly thicker than normal pancakes. Cook for 2 to 3 minutes on each side.

Entree Recipes

Salmon & Roasted Asparagus w/ Lemon & Caper Sauce

This recipe is a light, simple and clean. The flavors of the sauce compliment both salmon and asparagus nicely. It is very easy and perfect for an everyday meal or a dinner party if you choose to have one. Makes 4 servings.

Ingredients

- 2 tbsp lemon juice
- 2 tbsp shallots, minced
- 1 ½ tbsp olive oil
- 1 ½ tbsp capers, drained and chopped
- 1 tsp fresh thyme, chopped
- ½ tsp lemon zest, finely grated
- 1 ½ lbs skinless salmon fillet
- 1 lb asparagus spears, trimmed
- sea salt and pepper to taste

Directions

1. In a small bowl, whisk together lemon juice, shallots, 1 tbsp olive oil, capers, thyme and lemon zest.
2. Season with salt and pepper.
3. Preheat oven to 450 degrees.

4. Cut three ½ inch deep slits crosswise in the top of the salmon fillets as if you were dividing each fillet into four portions, just do not cut all the way through.
5. Coat asparagus spears in ½ tbsp olive oil and arrange in a single layer on a baking tray. Sprinkle with salt and pepper.
6. Place salmon on top of asparagus spears. Season with salt and pepper.
7. Gently spoon sauce over salmon and asparagus.
8. Roast until salmon is just starting to turn opaque in the center, about 20 minutes.
9. Divide into four portions, serve and enjoy!

Pecan-Rosemary Crusted Tilapia

Tilapia is a great source of selenium which is needed to allow the body to use phytonutrients that help to improve inflammation symptoms. This recipe is simple enough to make for a weeknight dinner with the family but can also be used for a dinner party. You can also use trout or cod for this recipe if you prefer. Makes 4 servings.

Ingredients

- ⅓ c raw pecans, soaked, dried and chopped
- ⅓ c panko breadcrumbs
- 2 tsp fresh rosemary, finely chopped
- ½ tsp granulated Stevia
- ⅛ tsp sea salt
- pinch of cayenne pepper

- 1 ½ tsp olive oil
- 1 egg white
- 1 lb tilapia fillets (4 oz each)

Directions

1. Preheat oven to 350 degrees.
2. In a small baking dish, combine pecans, breadcrumbs, Stevia, salt and cayenne pepper.
3. Add olive oil and toss to combine.
4. Bake pecan mixture until golden brown, about 7 minutes.
5. Increase oven heat to 400 degrees.
6. Spray a large glass baking dish with cooking spray.
7. In a shallow dish, whisk egg white until frothy. Dip fillet in egg white and then pecan mixture. Be sure to coat both sides.
8. Place fillets in prepared baking dish.
9. Press any remaining pecan mixture into tops of fillets.
10. Bake about 10 minutes. Serve hot.

Turkey & Quinoa Stuffed Peppers

This recipe gives the 1950s classic a modern twist. Sweeter red, yellow or orange peppers and using quinoa instead of calorie heavy, inflammation inducing breadcrumbs make it a much lighter dish. Makes 6 servings.

Ingredients

- 3 large yellow, orange or red bell peppers

- 1 ¼ lb ground turkey
- 1 tbsp olive oil
- 1 c mushrooms, chopped
- 1 c yellow onion, diced
- 2 tsp fresh garlic, minced
- 1 c tomato sauce
- 1 c chicken stock
- 1 c uncooked quinoa
- ½ c Parmesan, shaved

Directions

1. In a small saucepan, cook quinoa according to package directions.
2. In a large skillet, saute onions until translucent.
3. Add garlic. Saute until fragrant.
4. Add mushrooms and cook until softened.
5. Add ground turkey. Cook over medium heat until mostly cooked.
6. Add tomato sauce and ½ c of the chicken stock. Simmer until the turkey is fully cooked and the excess liquid has cooked away.
7. Preheat oven to 400 degrees.
8. Prepare peppers while turkey simmers. Wash them, cut in half, stem and seed them.
9. Spray a 9 x 12 baking dish with cooking spray and place peppers in the pan hollow side up.
10. Add quinoa to turkey mixture, stir to combine.
11. Divide quinoa/turkey mixture evenly between 6 pepper halves.

12. Top with just enough cheese to barely cover the stuffing.

13. Pour remaining chicken stock into baking dish for poaching peppers while cooking.

14. Cover dish with foil.

15. Bake for 30-35 minutes. Serve and enjoy!

Salad & Side Recipes

Tropical Quinoa & Cashew Salad

This salad is loaded with essential amino acids and is a great source of protein. It is very easy to make and has a creamy, nutty flavor that blends with almost any dish you choose to pair it with. Enjoy as a light meal or as a side dish. Makes 4 servings.

Ingredients

- 1 c uncooked quinoa
- ¼ c red onion, finely chopped
- 1 c apple, peeled, cored and finely chopped
- 2 tbsp lime juice
- 2 tbsp raw honey
- 1 tbsp olive oil
- 1 large mango, peeled, seeded and chopped
- ¼ c fresh mint, finely chopped
- sea salt and pepper to taste
- 1 tbsp fresh ginger, finely grated
- 1 Hass avocado, peeled, seeded and chopped or thinly sliced
- 1 c raw cashews, coarsely chopped
- 3 c Romaine lettuce, roughly chopped

Directions

1. Cook quinoa according to package instructions.
2. When cooked, spread out in an even layer to cool completely.
3. In a large bowl, whisk together lime juice, honey and olive oil.
4. Add onion and apple. Stir to coat.
5. Add cooled quinoa and mango. Toss well.
6. Add mint, cilantro and ginger. Salt and pepper to taste. Mix to combine.
7. Spoon mixture over Romaine to serve. Garnish with avocado and cashews.

Swiss Chard w/ Raisins & Almonds

This recipe is an easy and flavorful way to add chard to your menu. The toasted almonds contrast wonderfully with the savory, caramelized onions, sweet raisins and earthy chard. Makes 4 servings.

Ingredients

- 1 c yellow onion, thinly sliced
- 2 ½ tbsp olive oil
- 1 4/ tsp smoked paprika
- 2 lbs Swiss chard, discard ribs, washed and coarsely chopped
- ½ c golden raisins
- ¼ c water

- ¼ c raw almonds, sliced or slivered

Directions

1. In a heavy skillet, heat ½ tbsp olive oil over medium-low heat. Add almonds, stir frequently until golden, about 3 to 5 minutes.
2. In a dutch oven, heat remaining olive oil over medium heat.
3. Add onion and ¼ tsp salt. Saute until softened.
4. Add paprika and cook for 1 minute more, stirring constantly.
5. Add chard. Stir frequently until wilted.
6. Add raisins and water. Cook covered, stirring occasionally until chard is tender, about 7 minutes.
7. Season with salt and pepper.
8. Sprinkle almonds over chard and serve hot or cold.

Spinach & Goat Cheese Salad w/ Oregano Dressing

The combination of flavors in this salad pairs well with many entree choices. It may go best with dishes that need some lightening of flavors. This simple and delicious salad would go especially well with grilled lamb or steak. Makes 4 servings.

Ingredients

- 2 tbsp olive oil
- 2 tbsp lemon juice

- 1 tbsp Dijon mustard
- 1 tsp raw honey
- 1 tbsp fresh oregano, finely chopped
- 3 c baby spinach leaves
- 1 c red bell pepper, seeded and diced
- ½ c celery, thinly sliced
- ¾ c goat cheese, crumbled
- ⅓ c red onion, chopped
- sea salt and pepper to taste
- your choice of toasted pecans, almonds or pine nuts for garnish (opt)

Directions

1. Whisk together first 5 ingredients and ½ c goat cheese until well combined. Season with salt and pepper.
2. Add bell pepper, celery and onions to dressing. Toss to coat.
3. Add spinach. Toss to combine, spinach should be lightly coated with dressing.
4. Add remaining cheese. Garnish and serve

.

Kale & Chicken Caesar Salad

A great way to use up leftover roasted chicken is to add it to salads. These are perfect for a lunch on the go since the salad can be rolled into a wrap and taken to eat on the way to work or to put into your kid's lunch box. Makes 2-4 servings.

Ingredients

- 1 c grilled chicken, thinly sliced
- 6 c kale, discard ribs, washed and chopped
- 1 c cherry tomatoes, quartered
- ¾ c Parmesan cheese, shaved
- 1 egg, hard-boiled and chopped
- 1 tsp fresh garlic, finely minced
- ½ tsp Dijon mustard
- 1 tsp raw honey
- 2 tbsp lemon juice
- 3 tbsp olive oil
- sea salt and pepper to taste

Directions

1. In a large bowl, whisk together garlic, mustard, honey, lemon juice and olive oil. Whisk until thick and creamy. Season with salt and pepper to taste.
2. Add egg, chicken and tomatoes. Toss to coat with the dressing.
3. Add kale and Parmesan. Gently toss to combine.
4. Serve as a salad or spoon into a wrap.

Roasted Root Vegetables

While this recipe concentrates on root vegetables, it is very forgiving on the types of vegetables used in it. The combination of onion, garlic and rosemary gives the vegetables a lovely fragrance and a savory flavor. Makes 6-8 servings.

Ingredients

- 5 c butternut squash, peeled, seeded, cubed into ½ inch pieces
- 2 c beets (golden and red), trimmed, scrubbed, cubed into ½ inch pieces
- 2 yellow onions, quartered
- 1 c turnip, peeled, cubed into ½ inch pieces
- 1 c carrot, peeled, cut into ½ inch pieces
- ½ c fresh garlic, peeled and finely minced
- 2-3 tbsp olive oil
- 2 tbsp fresh rosemary, finely chopped
- sea salt and pepper to taste

Directions

1. Preheat oven to 400 degrees.
2. Oil 2 baking trays.
3. Combine all ingredients in a very large bowl. Toss to coat all vegetables in olive oil.
4. Spread vegetables on baking trays in an even layer. Season with salt and pepper.

5. Roast vegetables until tender and golden brown, about 1 hour. Stir occasionally to keep from burning.

6. Serve hot or make ahead and rewarm in 350 degree oven for 15-30 minutes.

Shiitake Mushrooms & Pea Pods

The earthy flavor of Shiitake mushrooms combine delightfully with sweet, crunchy pea pods in this dish. It makes a good accompaniment with fish and goes with most grains as well.

Ingredients

- 1 lb sugar snap peas
- ½ lb fresh Shiitake mushrooms
- 3 tsp toasted sesame oil
- 2 tsp granulated Stevia
- ¼ c dry sherry
- 2 tbsp natural soy sauce

Directions

1. Trim ends and any strings from pea pods. Trim stems from mushrooms and either discard or save for vegetable stock.

2. Slice mushrooms into ½ inch width pieces.

3. In a large skillet, heat sesame oil over medium-high heat.

4. Add mushrooms and saute until mushrooms just start to brown.

5. Sprinkle with Stevia and add sherry and soy sauce.

6. Cook and stir for 1 minute.

7. Add pea pods. Cook for about 2 minutes until peas are bright green and tender but crunchy.

8. Remove cover and continue to cook until most of the liquid evaporates.

9. Serve hot.

Soup & Curry Recipes

Red Lentil & Squash Stew

This is a really good soup to make ahead of time. You can portion it out into single servings, freeze it and take it with you anywhere. Just pop it in the microwave when lunchtime rolls around and you've got a savory, filling meal to keep you going until supper time. Makes 4 servings.

Ingredients

- 1 tsp olive oil
- 1 yellow onion, chopped
- 3 cloves garlic, finely minced
- 1 tbsp curry powder
- 4 c chicken broth
- 1 c red lentils
- 3 c butternut squash, steamed to tenderness
- 1 c baby spinach, packed
- 1 tsp fresh ginger, finely grated
- sea salt and pepper to taste

Directions

1. In a dutch oven, heat olive oil over medium-low heat. Add onion and garlic. Saute for about 5 minutes until fragrant and softened.
2. Add curry powder. Stir well and cook 1 additional minute until fragrant.

3. Add broth and lentils. Increase heat until mixture boils. Reduce heat to medium and simmer 10 minutes.

4. Add squash and spinach. Continue cooking for 8 minutes.

5. Season with salt, pepper and ginger to taste.

Black Bean Soup

Beans are an inexpensive and are packed with fiber, protein, folic acid, potassium and magnesium. This recipe takes a while to make so you might want to make it ahead of time and reheat as you want to serve it. The earthy flavor of the black beans takes on a new component when you combine it with onion, garlic and cumin. You can brighten it up with a splash of lemon juice if you desire though this recipe does not include that ingredient. Makes 4-6 servings.

Ingredients

- 1 c dried black beans
- 1 bay leaf, whole
- 1 yellow onion, chopped
- 2 cloves garlic, finely minced
- ½ tsp ground cumin
- ½ c dry sherry

Directions

1. Pick over the beans, removing dirt, stones or other foreign objects. Wash beans in clean water until water runs clear. Soak beans for at least 8 hours in lots of cold water.
2. Drain beans, rinse and then cover with fresh water. Bring to a boil over high heat with the bay leaf. Skim off any foam that rises to the top. Lower heat to medium-low, partially cover and simmer until beans are tender, about 1 hour.
3. Add onion. Continue to cook for 1 hour.
4. Add garlic. Season with salt and pepper to taste. Continue cooking until the skin of the beans split and the beans are very soft. This could take another 1-2 hours. Add more water as necessary.
5. Remove from heat and take out bay leaf.
6. Using a blender, food processor or immersion blender, puree until as smooth as it will get.
7. Return pureed soup to pan. Add cumin and sherry. Adjust seasoning as needed. Bring back to temperature over low heat before serving.
8. Garnish with lemon juice to taste and/or freshly chopped herbs as desired.

Chickpea & Broccoli Curry

The flavors in this dish blend so well together that you will fall in love with it. There is just enough chili bite to balance the creamy cashews with the delightful crunch of broccoli. Makes 4 servings.

Ingredients

- ⅓ c raw cashews, toasted
- 1 c water
- 1 tbsp coriander seeds
- 2 tsp cumin seeds
- 1 inch cinnamon stick
- 3 whole cloves
- 2 tbsp coconut oil
- 3 c yellow onion, diced
- 1 clove garlic, minced
- 1 tbsp fresh ginger, finely grated
- 1 tsp sea salt
- 1 tsp ground turmeric
- ½ – 1 tsp chili flakes
- 1 ½ c chickpeas, cooked
- 1 c tomatoes, chopped
- 3 c broccoli florets, cut into bite-sized pieces and steamed
- ½ c Greek yogurt
- cilantro, chopped for garnish

Directions

1. In a blender, combine cashews and water. Puree until smooth, about 30 seconds. Set aside for later use.
2. In a small skillet, add all whole spices and toast over medium heat until the seeds start to brown and smell fragrant. Allow to cool before grinding into a fine powder.

3. In a medium sized saucepan, heat oil over medium-high heat. Add onions, garlic, ginger and salt. Saute until onions are translucent, about 2 minutes.
4. Add turmeric, chili flakes, chickpeas and ground spice mixture. Saute for 2 minutes.
5. Reduce heat to low. Stir in cashew liquid. Simmer for 2 minutes.
6. Add tomatoes and simmer for 5 minutes.
7. Add broccoli florets and yogurt. Stir to combine and simmer for 1-2 minutes.
8. Remove from heat, salt to taste. Serve over rice and garnish with cilantro.

Italian Stew

This recipe is perfect for using your garden surplus vegetables. It makes a hearty and filling meal through the summer and early fall when garden produce is at its peak. If you are allowing yourself a treat, make it crusty bread to go with this delicious stew or cook the stew down more to go with your favorite pasta dish. Makes 4 servings.

Ingredients

- 2 c eggplant, skin on and cut into 1 inch cubes
- 1 tbsp olive oil
- 1 yellow onion, thinly sliced
- 5 cloves garlic, finely minced
- 1 stalk celery, thinly sliced

- 1 c fresh basil, stemmed and chopped
- 5 plum tomatoes, peeled and finely chopped
- 3 medium sized sweet potatoes, scrubbed and cut into 1 inch cubes
- 2 c zucchini, peeled and cut into ½ inch half rounds
- 2 red or yellow bell peppers, seeded and cut into 1 inch pieces
- sea salt and pepper to taste

Directions

1. Toss together eggplant and 2 tsp salt to sweat out the bitterness. Allow to sit for 20-30 minutes. Rinse, drain and pat dry.
2. In a large pot, heat oil over medium-high heat. Add onion, garlic and celery. Saute for about 5 minutes. Add a little water as necessary to keep it from sticking and burning.
3. Add basil. Saute for 1 minutes.
4. Add tomatoes, eggplant, sweet potatoes and ½ tsp salt. Stir and bring to a boil.
5. Reduce heat and simmer covered for 15 minutes.
6. Add zucchini and peppers. Simmer for 15 minutes until all vegetables are tender.
7. Remove from heat. Season with salt and pepper to taste. Allow to sit for 15 minutes before serving.

VARIATION NOTES: You can try any kind of summer squash in place of the zucchini. Try adding cauliflower or fennel root. If you don't like eggplant, substitute your favorite mushrooms instead.

French Lentil Soup

There is nothing that warms you up more on cold, rainy days than a robust, Mediterranean inspired stew. This soup is thick with French lentils, sweet potatoes and mushrooms that will satisfy that need for something filling and comforting while still letting you enjoy your new lifestyle. Makes 8-10 servings.

Ingredients

- 2 c yellow onion, coarsely chopped
- 3 cloves garlic, finely minced
- 2 c Cremini mushrooms, thinly sliced
- 8 c vegetable or chicken stock
- 1 ½ c French lentils, rinsed
- 2 c sweet potatoes, washed and cubed into 1 inch pieces
- 1 c celery, coarsely chopped
- 2 tbsp fresh rosemary, minced
- 2 tsp fresh thyme, minced
- 3 bay leaves
- 1 tsp smoked paprika
- 1 tsp pepper
- 2 c tomatoes, chopped
- ¼ c red wine

Directions

1. In a soup pot, dry saute the onion and garlic on medium heat, about 2 minutes.

2. Add mushrooms. Saute for another 5 minutes. Ingredients will stick but don't worry about the stuff browning on the bottom (this is called fond), it adds flavor to the soup.

3. Add remaining ingredients except tomatoes and wine. Bring to a boil.

4. Cover and reduce heat. Simmer for 30 minutes.

5. Add tomatoes and wine. Simmer for 2 minutes.

6. Remove from heat and serve.

Dessert Recipes

Coconut Flan

This light tofu pudding is a lot like an egg custard made with coconut milk. If you are a fan of traditional flan, you will find this dish to be delicious and a healthy substitute for that creamy treat. If you don't tell your guests it's not traditional, they likely won't even know the difference. Makes 6 servings.

Ingredients for the Syrup

- 5 tbsp coconut sugar
- 3 tbsp water

Ingredients for the Pudding

- ⅔ c extra-firm silken tofu, crumbled
- 2 tbsp coconut sugar
- 1 tbsp syrup
- ¾ tsp coconut extract
- ⅛ scant tsp sea salt
- 2 ½ c coconut milk (substitute soy milk, rice milk or almond milk as desired)
- ¾ tsp powdered gelatin

Directions for Syrup

1. Bring water and sugar to a boil over low heat. Simmer uncovered for 5 minutes. Remove from heat.

Directions for Pudding

1. Place tofu, 1 tbsp syrup, 2 tbsp sugar, coconut extract and salt in a blender. Do not blend yet, set it aside until needed.
2. Divide remaining syrup into 6 custard molds. Rotate each mold to coat the bottom and sides with syrup. Set aside.
3. In the syrup pan, bring your choice of milk and gelatin to a boil quickly. Stir constantly.
4. Reduce heat and simmer for 5 minutes to allow to thicken. Continue stirring.
5. Add hot milk mixture to blender. Blend until smooth.
6. Gently stir until most of the bubbles are re-incorporated.
7. Pour blended mixture into coated molds. Skim off any foam that remains.
8. Cover molds with plastic wrap and refrigerate at least 1 hour before serving.

To unmold flan

1. Dip bottom of each mold briefly into boiling water above the level of the pudding.
2. Remove plastic wrap and turn upside down on a dessert plate.
3. Pour any excess syrup over the pudding.
4. Garnish with fruit or chiffenaded mint leaves.

Sesame Almond Cookies

You like cookies, don't you? Everyone loves some kind of cookie. Unfortunately most store bought cookies are filled with all kinds of unhealthy ingredients and man-made chemicals. These tasty cookies are made with olive oil, tofu and chopped almonds so they are perfect to enjoy with a nice hot cup of green tea. Makes 4 dozen.

Ingredients

- 1 ½ c almond flour
- 1 tsp baking powder
- ⅛ tsp salt
- ¼ c sesame seeds, toasted
- ¾ c raw almonds, coarsely chopped
- 4 oz silken tofu, crumbled
- ½ c olive oil
- ¾ c coconut sugar
- 1 tbsp almond extract

Directions

1. Preheat oven to 350 degrees.
2. In a bowl, sift together flour, salt and baking powder. Add sesame seeds and chopped almonds.
3. In another bowl, mix together tofu, olive oil, sugar and almond extract until well combined and mostly smooth.
4. Gently fold wet ingredients into the flour mixture.

5. Roll into 1 inch balls and gently flatten. Place on an ungreased baking sheet.

6. Bake for 10 minutes until edges begin to brown.

7. Remove from baking sheet and allow to cool on a rack.

Ginger Almond Pears

This recipe has a lot of uses; you can use it to top your favorite vegan ice cream, add it to oatmeal to liven up your breakfast, enjoy it hot or cold as a compote or applesauce. The ginger in this dish gives the pears a special zing to wake up your tastebuds. Makes 6 servings.

Ingredients

- 5 firm, ripe pears; Barlett, Anjou, Bosc or your favorite
- 3 c apple cider
- 2 tsp fresh ginger, finely grated
- 3 tbsp arrowroot powder
- ⅓ c water
- ½ tsp almond extract
- sea salt to taste

Directions

1. Peel and core pears. Slice thinly and place in saucepan with apple cider and grated ginger. Add pinch of salt.

2. Bring to a boil. Reduce heat to medium-low and simmer until pears are tender, about 15 minutes.

3. Dissolve arrowroot powder in water. Add to simmering pears. Stir constantly until thick and clear.

4. Remove from heat. Stir in almond extract.

5. Serve warm or cold.

Apple Cake Squares

The best thing about this cake is that it is so easy to make! It's a moist cake and has a wonderful cinnamon-apple flavor. Serve it for dessert, as a quick and handy breakfast or take it in your lunch to school or work. Makes 9 servings.

Ingredients

- 1 c coconut flour
- ¼ tsp sea salt
- ¾ tsp nutmeg
- 1 tsp baking soda
- 1 tsp cinnamon
- 3 tbsp coconut sugar
- 3 tbsp butter, softened
- 2 eggs
- 2 c apples, peeled, cored and shredded
- ¼ c dates, finely chopped

Directions

1. Preheat oven to 350 degrees.

2. Sift together flour, salt, nutmeg, baking soda and cinnamon together in a medium sized bowl.

3. Cream together butter and sugar in another bowl.

4. Beat in eggs and whisk until smooth and creamy.

5. Stir in apples and dates until well mixed.

6. Stir dry ingredients slowly into wet ingredients to create batter.

7. Spray bottom and sides of 9 inch square baking dish with nonstick cooking spray.

8. Bake cake for 45 minutes.

9. Remove from oven and allow to cool before cutting.

10. Serve warm or at room temperature.

Lemon Ginger Sorbet

When you are really wanting ice cream to ease the heat of deep summer, try this healthy alternative. It has a tangy flair that will satisfy your sweet tooth and leave you feeling good about your indulgence. Serve with fresh fruit or mint leaves instead of the traditional ice cream toppings. Makes 6 servings.

Ingredients

- 1 c coconut sugar
- 1 tsp fresh ginger, finely grated
- 2 c Greek yogurt
- 1 ½ c coconut milk
- ½ c + 2 tbsp lemon juice
- 1 tsp lemon zest, finely grated

Directions

1. Stir together coconut milk and 2 tbsp lemon juice. Allow to sit for 10-15 minutes until milk curdles.
2. Combine all ingredients in a large bowl.
3. Refrigerate until thoroughly chilled.
4. Pour liquid into ice cream machine.
5. Run machine until frozen.
6. Serve immediately. Store leftovers in freezer.

Smoothie & Shake Recipes

Chocolate-Banana Shake

This shake brings back the memory of frozen bananas on a stick coated in chocolate. This is a much healthier version of that summertime snack that can be made in next to no time. Feel free to improvise by adding different flavors. Leftovers will keep for a week or two in the freezer. Makes 6 servings.

Ingredients

- 4 over-ripe bananas, peeled and frozen
- 2 tbsp unsweetened cocoa powder
- 1 tsp vanilla extract
- 2 tbsp coconut sugar

Directions

1. Place bananas in a blender or food processor. Pulse a few times to break up.
2. Add cocoa powder. Pulse to combine.
3. Add vanilla extract and sugar.
4. Blend until very smooth. Pour into glasses to serve immediately or into an air tight container to store in the freezer.

Green Protein Drink

Protein drinks often get a bad wrap for tasting nasty or being full of supposedly healthy ingredients that really aren't. However, green smoothies are all the rage! Well, guess what? This drink combines all the good things about protein drinks and green smoothies with none of the bad things. Nourish your body and boost your energy with this nutrient- and antioxidant-packed drink filled with plant-based protein. Makes 2 servings.

Ingredients

- 1 ½ c almond milk
- 1 large banana
- 1 c kale, ribs removed and thoroughly washed
- 5 dates, pitted
- 1 tbsp chia powder

Directions

- Combine all ingredients in a blender.
- Blend on high until smooth. Chia seeds may resemble the texture of tapioca.
- Divide into 2 glasses and enjoy!

-

Pineapple Almond Shake

The almonds give this invigorating shake a lot of protein. Light and fresh, this shake isn't difficult or time consuming to make for a quick end of the day snack or even something to start your day. If you don't care for almonds, try it with pecans or macadamia nuts instead. Makes 3 servings.

Ingredients

- ¼ c almonds, blanched and ground to powder
- 1 c fresh pineapple, roughly chopped
- ½ c ice, crushed or cubes
- ½ tsp coconut sugar
- ¼ c almond milk
- ½ c pineapple juice

Directions

1. Add all ingredients to a blender.
2. Puree until smooth.
3. Pour into 3 glasses and serve.

Summer Melon Soup

This is a sweet and silky melon soup that captures the essence of summer while the jalapenos give it a little kick. It's also a very versatile dish that is good for more than just dessert. Serve it as a cool entree or appetizer. For a bit more protein, add a quarter cup of lump crab meat to make it a whole meal on its own. Makes 6 servings.

Ingredients

- 4 c cantaloupe, cut into 1 inch pieces

- 4 c watermelon, cut into 1 inch pieces
- 3 tbsp lemon juice
- 2 tsp coconut sugar
- ¼ tsp sea salt
- 2 fresh jalapeno peppers, seeded and finely minced
- ½ c fresh blueberries

Directions

1. In a food processor or blender, liquefy cantaloupe and watermelon in batches. Transfer liquid to a bowl.
2. In last batch of melon, add remaining ingredients and puree.
3. Combine all liquified ingredients. Cover with plastic wrap and refrigerate for 4 hours or more before serving.

Conclusion

Now that you're through the entire mechanics, meal planning and core concept of DASH diet, it is time to apply your knowledge and witness the improvement in your life.

If you're actively fighting hypertension or other medical comorbidities such as diabetes mellitus, cardiovascular issues and electrolyte disturbances, this diet will prove miraculous to you in no time. All you have to do is commit yourself to eating well by focusing on this diet's main pointers, and gradually shifting towards a worthwhile and fun eating style.

Once you set your foot into starting a DASH diet, you will find utmost pleasure and enjoyment in eating tastier and healthier that you will certainly not think of leaving this diet plan for your lifestyle. There are hardly any restrictions on the tasty food in DASH diet and hence is the best diet plan that covers all aspects of health.

Use this eBook as a DASH diet guide in knowing all about DASH diet, the benefits, basics and implementing the diet in your life. Also, the most important part that is the actual diet plan should be followed properly, although you can make your own changes and do daily experiments in meals and recipes.

Also Consider Other Bestselling Dieting Books!

Check Out My Other Dieting Books!

Below you'll find some of my other dieting books that are popular on Amazon and Kindle as well. I'd love to show you all the different methods to losing weight and becoming healthy I have studied and written about, so you might learn which you prefer and find out works best for you.

All of them have been well received, and thousands of customers have achieved great results from the programs and the recipes in the book. Simply click on the links below to check them out. The next pages are brief previews of the books.

Vegan Diet

Coconut Oil

DASH Diet

Paleo Diet

Mediterranean Diet

Ketogenic Diet

Preview of Vegan Diet

Use the recipes of a vegan diet to build the body of your dreams and get the healthiest state of your life by applying the techniques and tips revealed within the book to transition into and stick with the vegan lifestyle

Vegan diet is a plant based diet which includes all the vegetables, fruits, nuts, greens, grains and all other food obtained from plants. It is low in saturated fats and high in carbohydrates and natural sugar (fructose).

Vegan diet is considered as one of the healthiest and balanced diet. Studies have shown that vegan diet or plant based diet has all the essential nutrition required by human body. There could be many reasons behind a person becoming vegan. Some reasons are related to religion, ethics and some are related to health and love for animals.

We are going to see all the superfoods which provide essential nutrients in vegan diet such as fat, proteins, calcium, iron, vitamins, zinc etc. Also, how you can transition to become a vegan from your current lifestyle and stick to this healthy diet without much efforts. I am going to show some of the healthy vegan recipes which are balanced in nutrients and also filling.

Check out the full book here

Or go to http://amzn.to/22bgxUm

Preview of Coconut Oil

Coconut oil is derived from coconut fruit. Coconut oil has been an integral diet of the human species since time immemorial. For over 4000 years of documented history, coconut oil has been used extensively by communities in tropical lands especially those along the shores of major water bodies such as oceans, seas and lakes.

The Coconut tree is one of the popular trees found along the tropical coastlines in Asia, Africa, Southern Europe, South America and several other parts of the world. It is one of the most versatile trees when it comes to its uses. It has been traditionally used for shelter as a building material, as food, as oil for cooking, as oil for skin beauty, as medicine, as detoxifying agent, as anti-microbial agent, among many other uses. Indeed, there is no part of the coconut tree that has no use. In this book we will learn how to use the variety of uses to our advantage and especially the multitude of ways we can use the oils of the coconut.

Check out the full book here!

Or go to http://amzn.to/1VNgJ72

Preview of DASH Diet

DASH means Dietary Approaches to Stop Hypertension. The DASH diet is a deep rooted way to deal with healthy eating that is intended to help treat or avoid (hypertension). The DASH diet urges you to lessen the sodium in your diet and eat an assortment of nourishment, rich in supplements that help lower blood pressure, for example, potassium, calcium and magnesium.

Similar to Vegan Diets, the DASH eating plan has been demonstrated to lower blood pressure in only 14 days, even without bringing down sodium consumption. Best reaction came in individuals whose blood pressure was just respectably high, incorporating those with pre-hypertension. For individuals with more extreme hypertension, who will most likely be using prescribed medicines, the DASH diet can enhance their compliance to drugs, and lower blood pressure with a natural approach too. The DASH diet can bring down cholesterol, and with weight reduction and activity, can decrease insulin resistance and diminish the risk of creating diabetes.

Check out the full book here!

Or go to http://amzn.to/1Xp0OL4

Preview of Paleo Diet

Carve out the body of your dreams with the strategies, techniques, and recipes revealed within for everything you need to know about going Paleo like a Pro!

The Paleo diet has been called the cousin of the ketogenic diet since both lifestyles promote a high fat, moderate protein, low carbohydrate intake of macronutrients. It is promoted as a way of improving your health because it reduces the amount of sugar that is converted into fat when it's not used right away. Most foods, including some meats, include carbohydrates so when your diet is full of grains and processed foods, this is a good thing.

The idea for this diet has been traced to a 1975 book by Walter Voegtlin who was a gastroenterologist. In 1985, it was further developed by Stanley Boyd Eaton and Melvin Konner. However, it didn't come into true popularity until 2002 when Dr. Loren Cordain published his book, The Paleo Diet.

If you are looking for a way to improve your own health, whether you want to lose weight or not, have more energy and just plain feel better then the Paleo diet may just be the one for you. Even if it's not the lifestyle you want to follow for the rest of your life, just 30 days will show you the value inherent in changing your eating habits to match our ancient ancestors.

Check out the full book here

Or go to http://amzn.to/1XnrMlL

Preview of Mediterranean Diet

You may have seen commercials touting the benefits of a Mediterranean diet cookbook and wondered if it really works. Well, if you are looking for a heart-healthy diet then the Mediterranean diet may be the right one for you. As with all diets, just limiting what and how much you eat isn't going to help you achieve your goals all on its own. That is what the Mediterranean diet is all about.

The Mediterranean diet cookbook is full of healthy fats, whole grains, seafood, legumes as well as fresh fruits and vegetables. You can even have moderate amounts of wine while following this diet. While eating fruits, vegetables, fish and whole grains while limiting unhealthy fats are part of all tried and true diets, subtle variations in the amounts you eat may make a difference in your risk of heart disease. This is why the Mediterranean diet has been determined to be one of the best and healthiest ways to eat. Thankfully, it is as good for your taste buds as it is for your health.

The Mediterranean diet emphasizes eating plant-based foods such as fresh fruits and vegetables, whole grains, legumes and nuts. The information in this book will show you how you can replace the unhealthy fats in oils you are currently consuming with healthy fats like olive oil and avocados. You'll see how using herbs and spices can make your meals taste even better than if you'd piled on the salt. While red meat is restricted, fish and poultry graces your plate a bit more often. It really is a diet worth your time. Making the may take some effort on your part, but if you make that effort you will soon be on the path toward a healthier lifestyle, a better body, more energy, and a longer life!

Check out the full book here

Or go to http://amzn.to/1Uclh7k

Preview of Ketogenic Diet

The ketogenic diet is closely related to the paleo diet which also excludes carbohydrates. Unfortunately, today's diet consists of a high level of carbohydrates which causes significant changes in our health, which don't help in the slightest for diseases like diabetes. Carbohydrates are by far the most fattening ingredient in our diets.

The ultimate goal of following a low-carbohydrate ketogenic diet is to improve your heath by making your body burn ketones rather than glucose for energy. Within this book you will learn what the ketogenic diet is and how it works, things you should know and do before starting this diet plan, and how to make it work for you.

By following a ketogenic diet, you can feel good in your own skin again! You'll have more energy, your skin and hair will be smoother and healthier, not to mention the reduction of stress, depression and anxiety that can nag you as you go about your day.

Check out the full book here!

Or go to http://amzn.to/1TG9G0E

www.ingramcontent.com/pod-product-compliance
Lightning Source LLC
Chambersburg PA
CBHW071235280526
45787CB00002B/936